10 Powerful Tips to Improve Lymph Flow

10 Powerful Tips to Improve Lymph Flow
Copyright (C) 2023 Laurel West, LMT

Contact Information:
www.LaurelwestLMT.com

Editorial assistance: Noelle McBride
Design Consulting: Kyle McBride

Paperback ISBN: 9798385786053

Written in the United States of America

This book is dedicated to all of my amazing clients, teachers, mentors and peers who have taught me so much on this never-ending journey of discovering the body, mind & spirit.

And to my sister, Noelle, who inspires me and has encouraged me to write my first book.

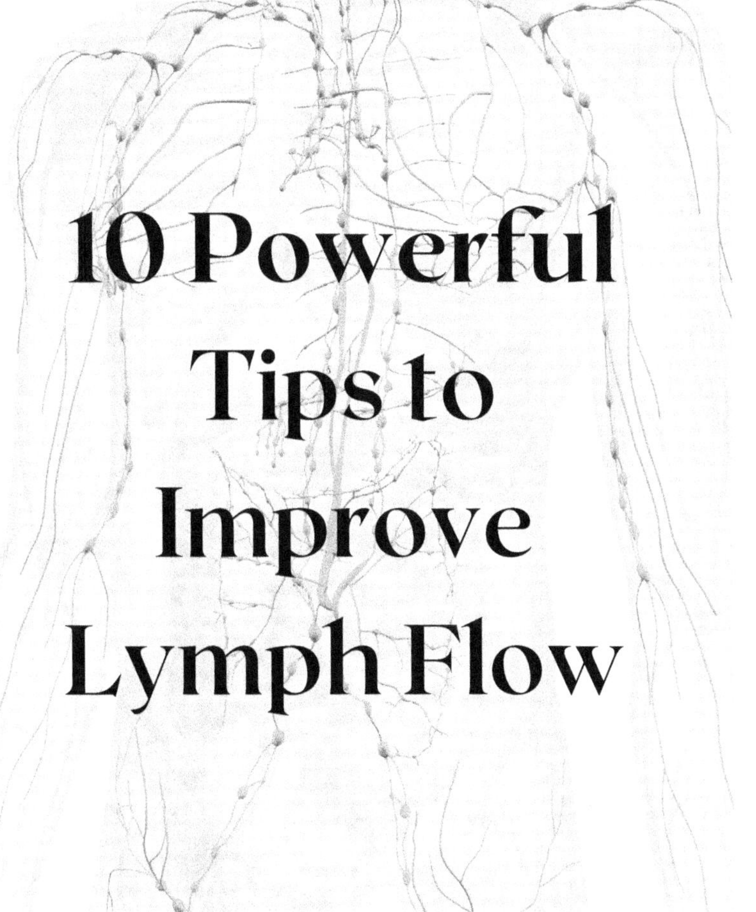

10 Powerful Tips to Improve Lymph Flow

Laurel West, LMT

Advanced Lymphatic Therapist

www.LaurelWestLMT.com

Sign up for the newsletter!

Receive announcements, latest news, printables, etc.

www.LaurelWestLMT.com

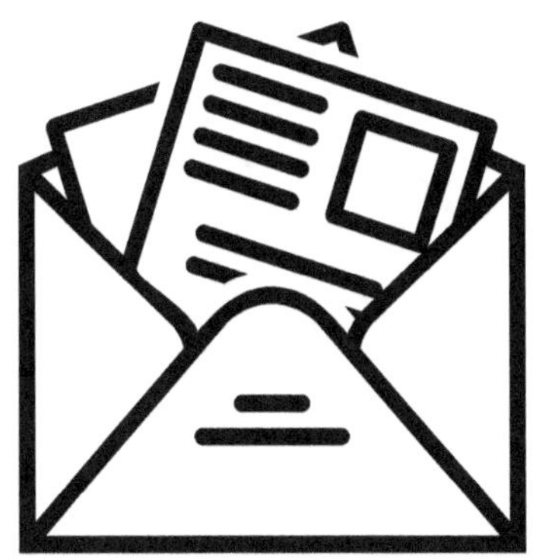

Table of Contents:

Introduction

Clients are always asking for tips to improve lymphatic health and these are the top ten that have been repeated like a broken record.

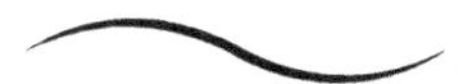

This book contains a brief overview of my top 10 tips. Individually, they are powerful in themselves, but combined, can be a game changer in optimizing your lymphatic health in as quickly as the first 30 days! Most importantly, you'll now have the tools to move your quality of life from surviving to thriving.
I always encourage my clients to do their own research and hopefully this book will help with a place to begin.

Disclaimer:

This is not a book about teaching manual lymphatic techniques, but rather, lymphatic lifestyle choices.

**Laurel West, LMT is not and does not claim to be an authority on any of the subject matter, nor a medical doctor, psychologist or licensed nutritionist and she recommends that any addition of herbs and supplements and/or change in your diet (and in some cases, receiving bodywork) be approved by your personal physician.

Listen to the sounds of
the waves within you.

RUMI

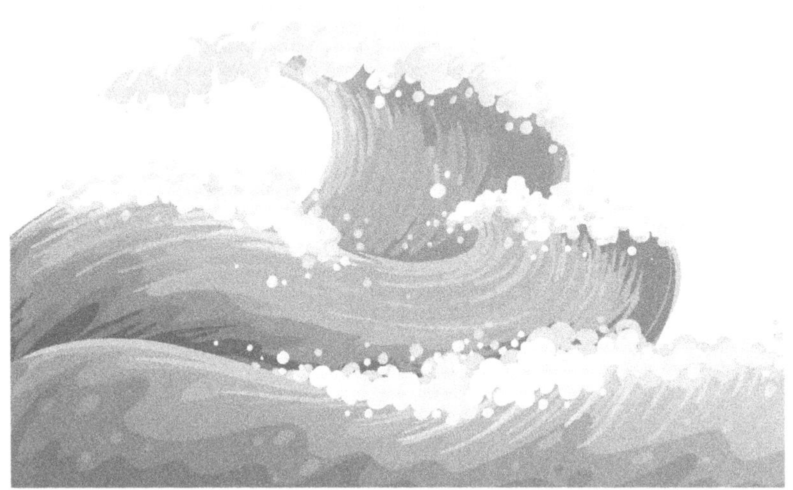

What is the Lymphatic System?

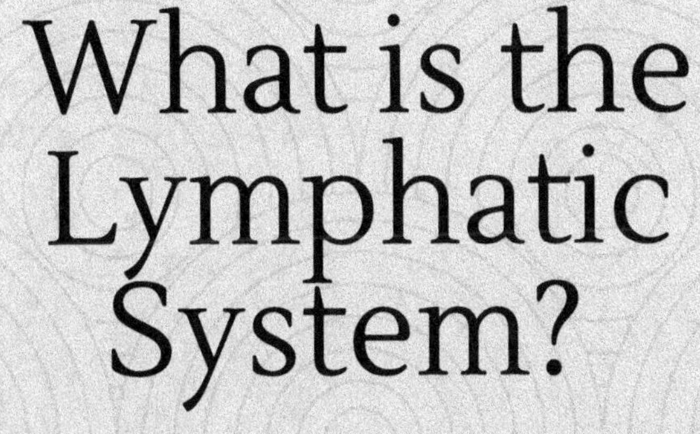

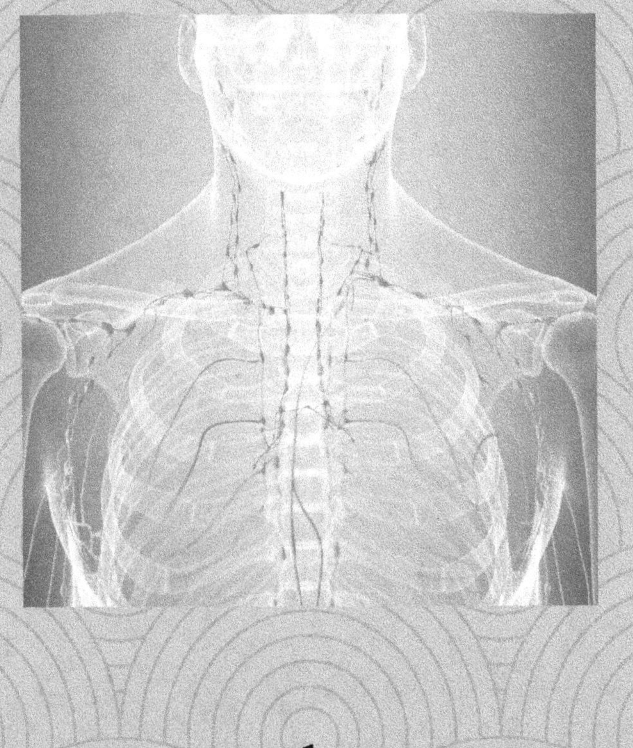

What is the Lymphatic System?

A brief overview

The lymphatic system is part of the immune system and helps the body fight disease. It keeps body fluid levels in balance, removes illness causing invaders, absorbs digestive tract fats and removes cellular waste.

The lymphatic system is made up of a network of lymph nodes, vessels, ducts and organs that carry lymph fluid from the body's tissues and returns it to the blood.

The lymph fluid contains nutrients & waste like white blood cells, fats and proteins. The lymph vessels are similar to blood vessels, but they carry lymph fluid instead.

The lymph nodes are small glands that filter & trap bacteria, viruses and other pathogens while the lymphocytes (white blood cells) destroys the diseases.

The human body can have anywhere From 400-800 lymph nodes that can be in clusters or chains throughout the body. The clusters that most people are aware of are in the neck, underarms & groin. These are the areas that most commonly will visibly swell due to the body fighting off an infection.

Lymphatic ducts return lymph to the bloodstream helping to maintain normal blood volume and pressure, as well as, preventing excess buildup of fluid in the tissues (edema).

Identifying a sluggish lymphatic system

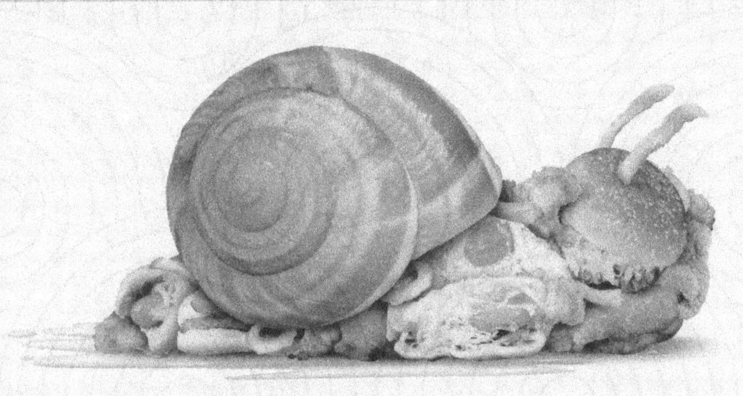

As a therapist, I can immediately feel when my client's lymph flow is sluggish. As soon as I sink my fingertips into the superficial waters of the lymphatic, it will at best feel like a pristine, flowing river of clean, clear water or, it can at times feel like; wading through a thick swamp or worse; like trying to push my fingers through cold molding clay or anywhere in between these polarities.

When our lymph feels like it's struggling to move, so does our entire being. In many cases, we can assist our bodies in flushing our internal toilets so to speak by incorporating small daily habits into our routines. Although, in other cases, we need all the tools in the toolbox and we may need the help of our therapists, doctors and specialists in addition to positive lymphatic lifestyle changes at home.

Embodying a level of self-awareness is also a key factor to identifying changes in our health. While this may be obvious to some, to many, it is not a state that they are familiar with. Ignoring or dismissing changes in our body, can be a form of self-abandonment and for whatever the reason may be, it can catch up with us! So if you're here reading this, I applaud you for now taking responsibility & action towards creating optimal health for yourself and/or loved ones.

The most common symptoms that clients schedule a visit with me are:

- Water retention, weight gain & puffiness
- Muscle stiffness & Joint pain
- Fatigue
- Sinus inflammation
- Headaches
- Dehydration
- Constipation, Bloating & Irritable bowel
- Swelling in extremities
- Overall feeling of sluggishness & lack of motivation
- Skin issues (acne, rashes, eczema, psoriasis)
- Allergies
- Digestive issues & inflammation
- Lung/Pleura inflammation & congestion
- Swollen lymph nodes
- Recovery from Infections/Disease
- Hormone Imbalances
- Female related issues (cysts, fibroids, pms, endometriosis)
- Pregnancy (fertility, post-partum)
- Auto-immune diseases
- Chronic inflammation
- Slow healing
- Post-surgery swelling
- Edema

How many of the tips in this book to include will depend on your individual health needs. If your lymph flow just needs a little boost, then you might consider just integrating a few of these tips into your routine. If your "river of life" has turned into a swamp land, then I recommend trying as many as possible on a consistent basis, with a loving dose of strong self-discipline.

Is your goal to maintain a healthy lymph system or to create one?
Did you find multiple symptoms on the list that you're experiencing?

If you're in an acute health crisis, you may want to start with adding a few gentle basics into your daily routine and then maybe work your way up to including multiple lymphatic boosters throughout the week.

Many of these tips are gentle enough for a healthy individual to add into a routine using their own discernment and intuition. In the cases of an acute health crises, please consider consulting your team of health professionals to assist and guide you safely through each addition or change that you consider making.

Lymph Flow Tip #1

DRINK YOUR WATER

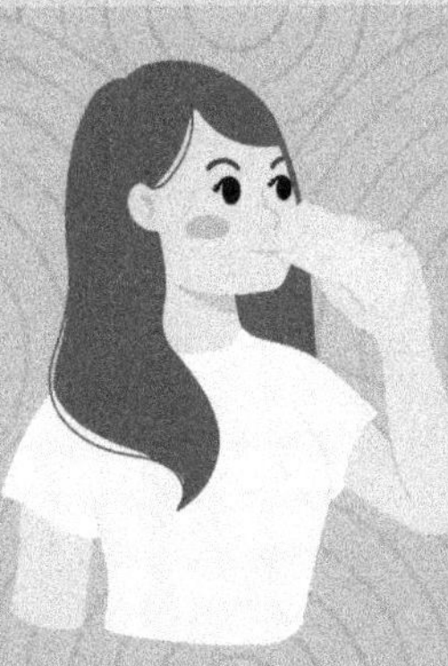

 Upon waking, our body needs fluids to assist in flushing out all of the metabolic waste that it has been working hard to collect throughout the night, during restorative sleep. I typically begin with 8oz of room temperature water to give my organs a gentle wake up.

I've always gone by the rule to take your body weight, divide it in half and that is at least how many ounces of water you should consume daily.

For example:
If you weigh 120 lbs, you should drink at least 60 oz of water per day. That being said, if you are sweating a lot during the day or drinking caffeine or taking other diuretics, you will need to increase your water intake.

An additional tip that I give is to invest in water purification for your home. If possible, whole home systems are available or you can opt for more affordable countertop options. Staying away from plastic water bottles is highly encouraged. Toxins & chemicals that can be leached into the water from plastics is an additional burden for the body to have to filter out through the lymphatic system and can have greater effects on our health than we realize.

One of my favorite analogies to share with my clients regarding the lymphatic system is comparing it to a toilet or sewage system. We all know that if the back of the toilet tank is not being refilled with fresh water, then there is nothing to flush the toxic sewage down the drain and therefore it will just sit and fester and create disease. GROSS!!

Second analogy is a vase of flowers. When we fail to change out the water in the vase frequently, the water gets cloudy, the stems get slimy and begin to break down. If we wait too long, the flowers wilt & die. Something similar happens when we allow toxic, old lymph fluid to remain stagnant in our tissues.

So, be sure to drink plenty of fresh, preferably purified water, to ensure your internal system can be flushed at all times.

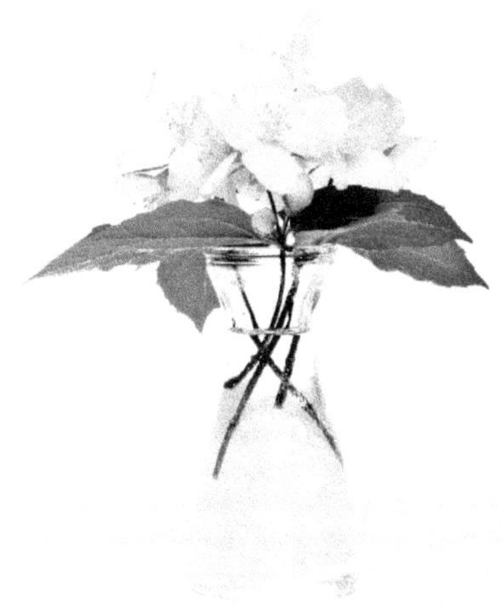

Lymph Flow Tip #2

MATCHA MEDITATION

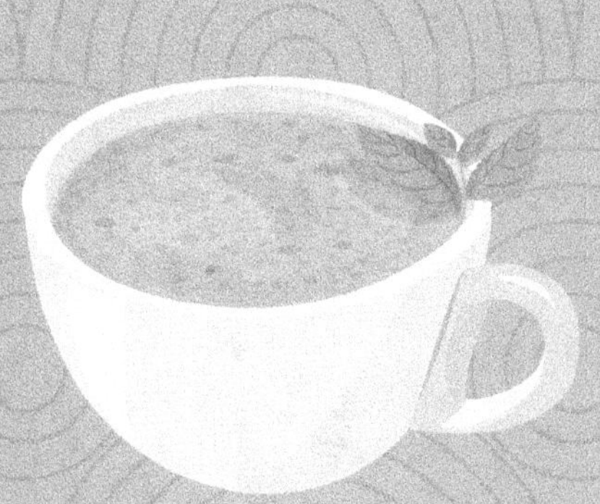

Notes

Matcha Meditation

While I was in my own personal detoxification/healing phase, I often made a hot, lemon-ginger matcha. This, to me, feels like an internal astringent, drawing out residual toxins and starting the day fresh & clean. It feels comforting, divine & pure.

I call it my Matcha Meditation.

Lemon-Ginger Matcha Recipe:

½ squeezed organic lemon (or lime)
1 tsp local raw honey
½ tsp organic ceremonial grade matcha powder
1 tsp freshly juiced or grated ginger (optional)
8oz purified hot water
1 Lemonbalm teabag (optional)
1 tsp Moringa powder (optional)

While waiting for the water to boil, squeeze lemon through a strainer into a mug, add honey & matcha and stir to make a vibrant green matcha paste. Slowly whisk in hot water and ginger, then add optional tea bag. Moringa powder is also a nice addition or substitute to the Matcha.

Let steep until you can comfortably hold your mug with both hands. Allow the warm steam to enter the sinuses, while you deeply inhale the smell of fresh spring. Sip slowly, feeling the magic you've created; cleanse, clear and awaken the body, mind & spirit. Ahhhhhhhh.

This act of presence & gratitude is the Matcha Meditation.
Namaste ;)

Lymph Flow Tip #3

BREATHWORK

There are many different methods of breathwork that are excellent. Find a method that resonates with you & your needs. I like to suggest that my clients check in with their bodies once an hour by taking 3-5 deep cleansing breaths, while being in awareness of where we're holding on to tension (ie: relaxing the jaw, shoulders, etc) and drinking some water. We can do this at our desk, at a stop light or most places during our day.

This type of breathwork stimulates the lymphatic system as your body expands & retracts. It activates the parasympathetic nervous system, calming the mind and body of anxiety & stress.

Other benefits include: (WebMD)

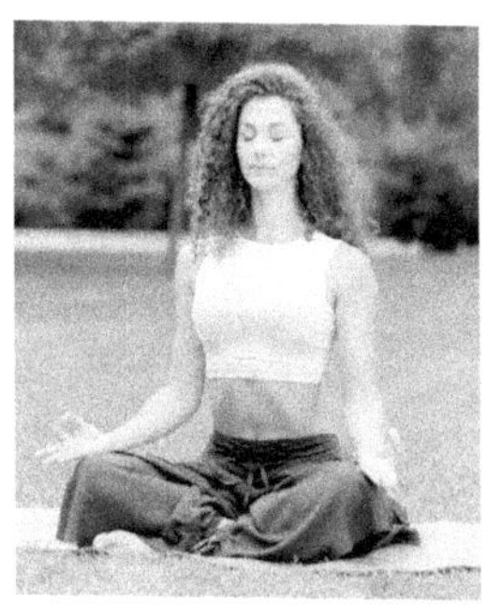

- Balanced blood pressure
- Improved sleep
- Strengthening lung function
- Better immune function
- Reduced feelings of PTSD & Trauma
- Release of stress hormones
- Anti-inflammatory effect
- Blood alkalizing
- Mood Elevating

My definition of a deep cleansing breath is to take a slow, long inhale through the nose, stretching and expanding out the ribcage, diaphragm and all the fascia surrounding it, hold that deep breath in for a second or two, then slowly exhale through the mouth or nose completely and repeat 3-5 times.

Lymph Flow Tip #4

DRY BRUSHING

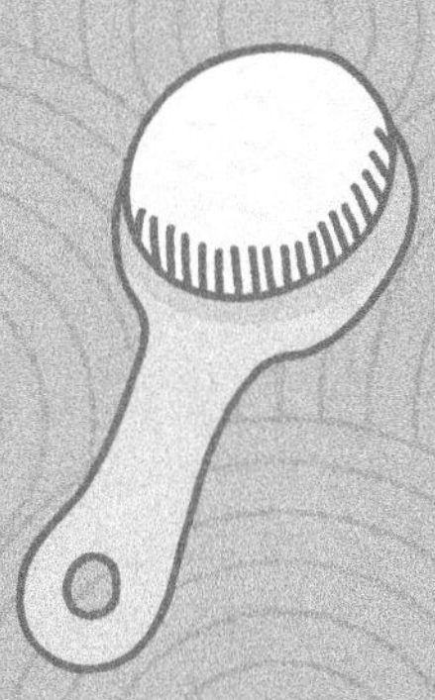

Dry Brushing

Using a dry brush is an excellent daily morning ritual to include before a workout or before we bathe to jumpstart our lymphatic detox.

Typically, a dry brush is either a short or long handled wooden brush with natural bristles. I prefer the short handle, because I feel I have better control of it and I can still reach the middle of my back, but it is whatever you prefer.

Like the name, you want to use this brush DRY, before entering the bath, shower, sauna, steam room or breaking a sweat. Each stroke is a flowing, yet brisk movement, making sure we cover the entire area of the skin.

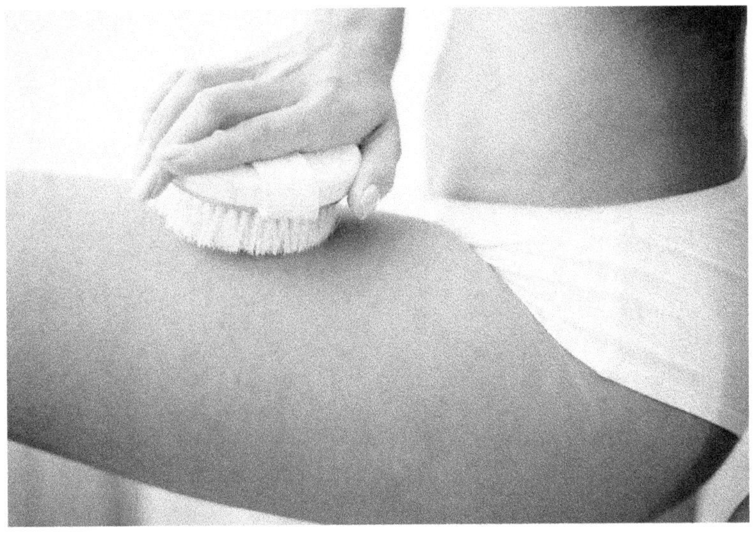

Remember:
We don't need to be perfect here.

This entire process should be a quick 5-10 minute ritual.
Dry brushing sloughs off dead skin cells and tones the skin, giving us that daily glow up!
It will also stimulate the lymph flow that may cause an invigorating feeling and even get the digestive system moving as well.

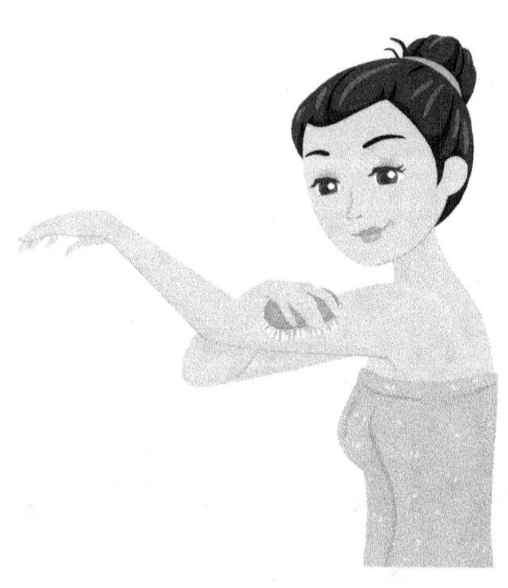

Dry Brushing

My personal routine:

Let's begin!

1. I start at the tops of my feet using small, quick strokes towards the ankles.
2. then move up my legs, with the length of the strokes from ankles to knees.
3. then knees to tops of thighs (towards the inguinal nodes, located at the top of our inner thighs).
4. Brush the front, back & all sides of our legs (excluding the genitals),
5. maybe giving a bit of extra attention to areas where we might collect more cellulite like the thighs & buttocks.
6. Then move to the abdomen. To make it quick and simple, I usually just stimulate this area with a clock-wise circular motion around the navel. If you are more experienced and want to get technical, then you can do smaller brush strokes towards the appropriate superficial nodes.
7. Next, I brush the arms all around from wrist towards axillary nodes (underarms).
8. Then I reach across to my flank area and brush upward from waist to underarms,
9. then from sternum, under each breast to under arms again. Next, above & around the breasts (being much more gentle on delicate skin like the décolletage, breasts, neck & face).
10. I personally do not dry brush my face or the front of my neck.
11. Then brushing downward on the back of my neck from the hairline, down neck and across the tops of my shoulders and to my collarbone.
12. For my back, I usually do circular motions everywhere I can reach.

And that's it. We are done!

27

Lymph Flow Tip #5

DETOX BATH RITUAL

Bathing is sacred and purifying to me and I believe should be treated as such. My bath typically lasts 15-30 minutes & 4x per week depending on my schedule. It's a time for being present & in full awareness of our bodies (physical, mental, emotional, energetic), for taking deep cleansing breaths, as well as, releasing tension and letting go of resistance.

There is no rule that bathtime is only for before bed. Many times, while I was experiencing a healing phase, my body was so stiff & sluggish, that I had to do my detox bath before anything else in order to have the ability to get moving for the day.

Hydration before, during and after a hot bath is important. Consult with your doctor first, especially if you have a history of heart related issues, dizziness, fertility issues or if you are pregnant.

Soaking in an epsom salt bath is not only excellent for stimulating the lymph system, cleansing skin & pores, it's also an excellent way to clear the energy body of unwanted debris. For this, salt is the key ingredient. I prefer Epsom salt for my baths and I save the Pink Himalayan Sea Salt for homemade salt scrubs that I use in the shower or to scrub my hands with in-between clients. For Epsom salt, I usually buy generic store brand and then I add 5-10 drops of whatever essential oil I'm drawn to for the day into at least 2 cups of epsom salt. I allow the essential oils to absorb into the salt while the bath is running, then pour the fragrant salt into the water once the bath is filled (I prefer a half full tub of warm-hot water) and then stir it around until the salt is dissolved.
Then ease in…. Ahhhhhhh.

During the 15 minutes of soaking, relaxing and bath time meditation, I'll usually fit in a few minutes of self lymphatic massage and deep breath work.

At the end of the bath, while the water is draining out, I like to use a cup to rinse off with fresh, clean water. If you're feeling brave, I highly recommend rinsing with uncomfortably cold water to simulate contrast therapy.

Then while my skin is still damp, I thoroughly massage organic body oil onto my entire body (I like pure organic almond oil), and then air dry or gently towel dry.

Other bath add-in items:

Mustard Bath powder
Pure Magnesium Flakes
Baking Soda
Bentonite clay
Ground oatmeal (for skin soothing)

Favorite essential oil blends for bath:

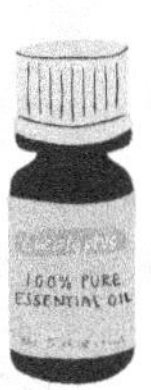
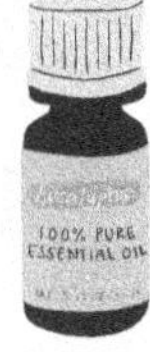

Orange & Peppermint
Geranium
Purify & Palo Santo
Bergamot & Rose
Lemon & Eucalyptus
Thieves or Guardian
Ginger & Lime

Lymph Flow Tip #6

STRETCH IT OUT

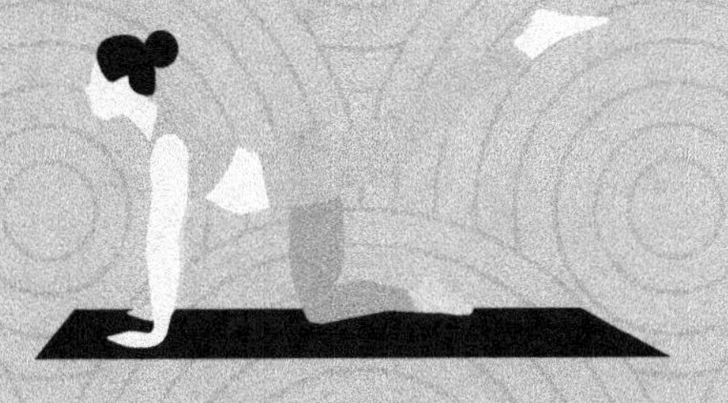

The lymph system is activated by a stretch & release response, unlike the circulatory system which uses the heart as a pump. Even the basic expansion and retraction of deep breathing stimulates some lymph movement. Lymphatic movement increases with walking and especially with intentional stretching. This stretching of the skin, fascia, muscles & organs is what is assisting our body to flush out that old lymphatic fluid.

Deep Yoga Yin stretching is a very effective and brilliantly designed method to move any stagnant energy in the body.

Get your body moving right away when you wake up. Gentle backward arm circles will activate all of the chains of lymph nodes around the breast, the axillary (underarm) region, clavicles, shoulders, etc. Walking around the house or around the block in the morning and/or even doing 5-10 minutes of basic stretching will assist lymph movement.

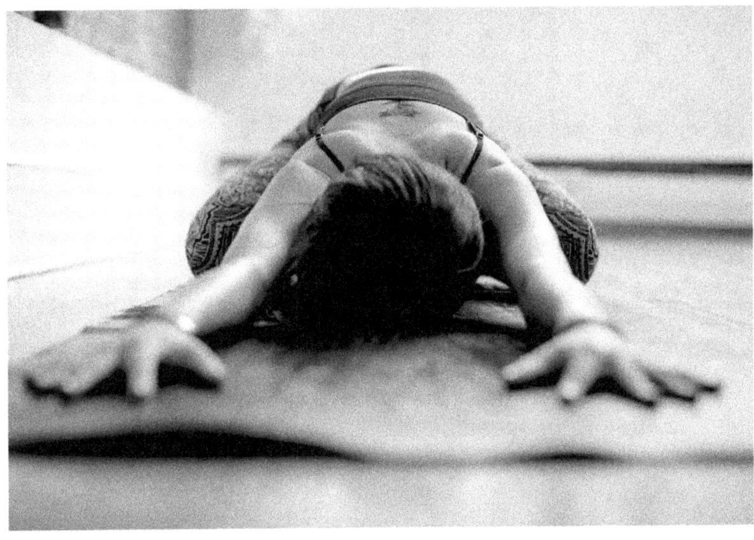

Lymph Flow Tip #7

SWEAT IT OUT

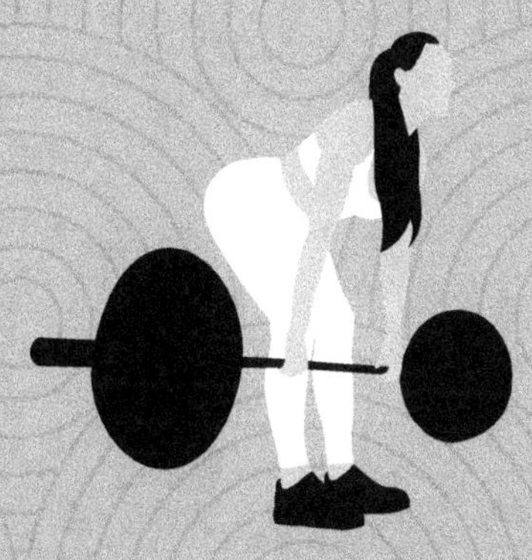

My morning gym routine (4-5x per week):

10-20 min walking on treadmill
10 min deep stretches
40 min weight lifting
10-20 min dry sauna

Sweat It Out

Sweating is another way the lymphatic system flushes out toxins. We can get creative on how to break that sweat.

Here's a few:

Detox baths
Infrared saunas
Steam room
Heated crystal mat with infrared
Cardio workouts
Weightlifting
Layer up on warm clothing

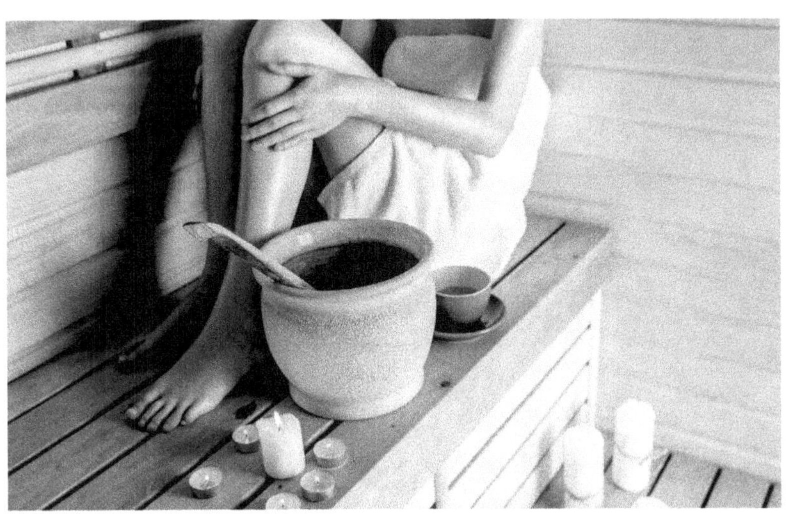

Lymph Flow Tip #8

LYMPHATIC FACIAL

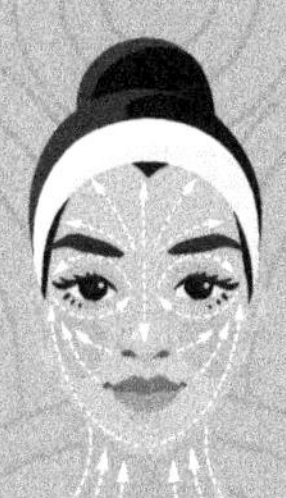

Lymphatic Facial

Lymphatic massage for the face can transform your appearance and skin health if done on a daily basis. Whether using your fingers, a tool or getting a professional lymphatic facial, it should all be very light touch. Gently sinking into the waters of the lymph with a pressure of only 5 grams (similar to the weight of a nickel on your skin). I suggest using a light facial oil on clean skin to maintain a feather light pressure and without pulling the skin. This type of massage feels fabulous at the end of a long day. I recommend getting a few professional lymphatic facials or watching some tutorial videos to perfect your at home facial.

Lymphatic massage benefits:

- Instant mini face lift (reduces appearance of folds & wrinkles)
- Helps release tension in the facial muscles
- Reduces puffiness
- Stimulates collagen production
- Detoxify skin
- Assists to clear up acne
- Drains the sinus cavities
- Extremely relaxing

Fun tools:
- Your hands (My fave)
- Jade rollers
- Cupping
- Gua Sha
- Dry brush for face

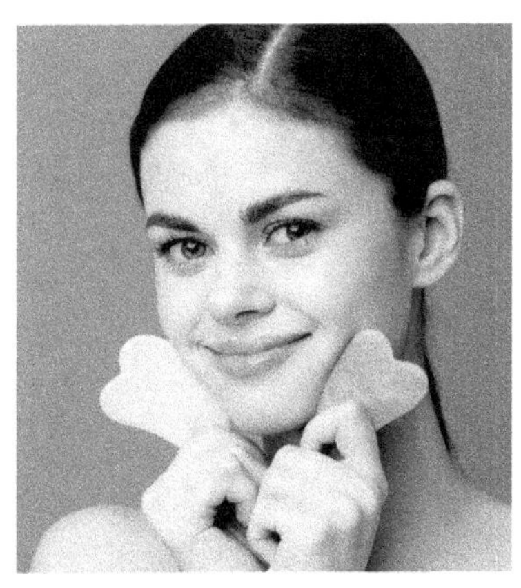

Lymph
Flow
Tip #9

ADVANCED LYMPHATIC MASSAGE

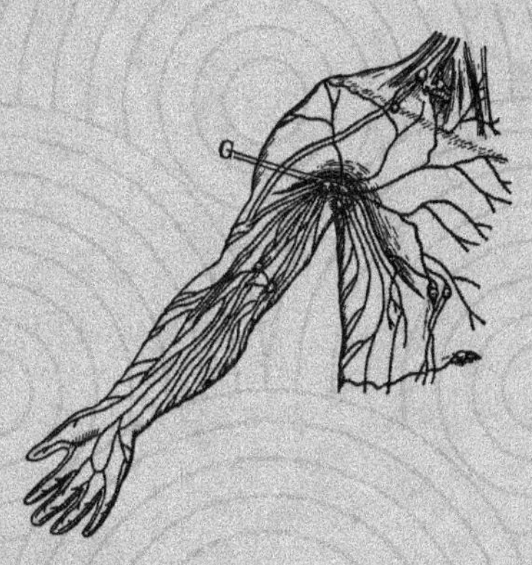

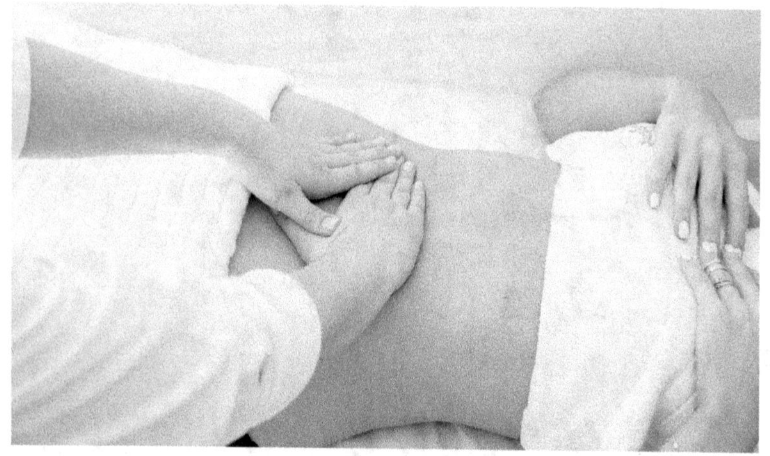

(photo credit: Carla Oliveira, Getty Images)

Advanced Lymphatic Massage for superficial lymph, deep abdominal nodes and viscera.

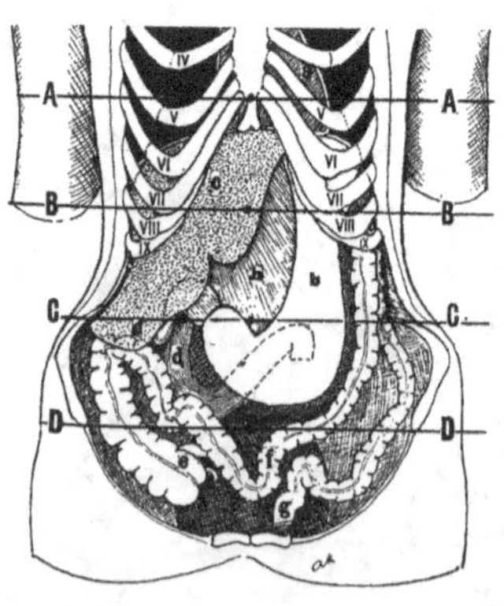

Lymphatic massage is a fantastic resource to jump start your journey to healthier lymph flow. Advanced lymphatic massage not only will move the superficial lymph that is skin deep, but also addresses all of the layers of the lymphatic of the body including the fascia, muscles, organs, brain (glymphatic), our deep lymphatic pathways, sinuses, digestion, down to the cellular level of our body.

In a typical advanced lymphatic session, the therapist will open up the superficial lymph nodes, as well as, the deep nodes in order to stimulate the nodes to begin pulling the lymph fluid towards the nodes like a vacuum. The practitioner then will move the lymph in the appropriate direction (lymphatic mapping is done to assess if the lymph fluid is moving where it should be). If an overall detox or flush is the goal, then a full body session will be done, including deep nodes and draining of the liver.

If the client has a specific need then the surrounding nodes will be opened then focused attention to the needed area. In cases where the specified area needs to be avoided, then the distal areas can be drained and can have a healing effect on the acute need.

Lymphatic massage frequency will differ for everyone and the individual needs. For acute issues, more frequent sessions may be required to achieve the best outcome. In all cases and especially acute issues and health crises, taking care of your lymphatic health at home in tandem with lymphatic massage sessions is key to optimal results.

Lymph Flow Tip #10

ANTI-INFLAMMATORY DIET

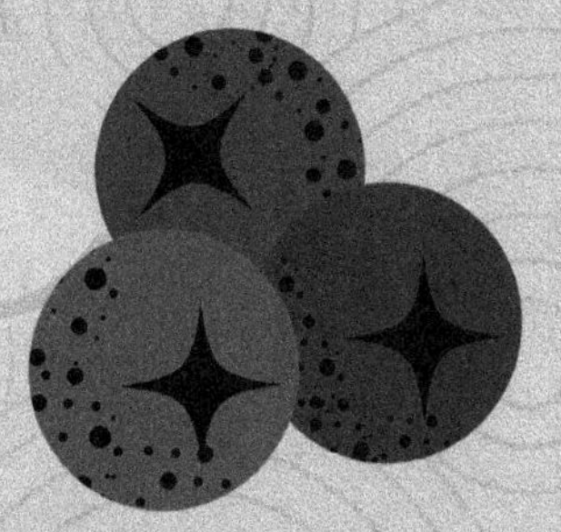

Frequently, I will recommend that my clients look into a 30 day elimination diet. The diet is widely known as the AIP diet (Auto-Immune Protocol). I like to refer to it as the Anti-Inflammatory Diet instead because it can be extremely beneficial for many inflammatory issues, outside of an auto-immune diagnosis. This tip is for those who are ready for a serious change.

The first phase is the elimination phase. This is when the highest inflammation causing foods are completely eliminated from our diet for a minimum of 30 consecutive days, up to a maximum 90 days. This allows for the body to fully detox and release these foods and to calm the sometimes chronic inflammation that they can cause so that the body is now out of that stressed state and able to begin a repair.

Second phase is reintroduction, where some or all of the items can be slowly reintroduced back into the diet to more easily be able to identify how those foods might trigger a reaction in our body and the way we feel.

The third phase of the protocol is the maintenance phase. Those who can remain committed for the entire protocol will have a diet created just for your body by the end of the journey!

The AIP diet is also an excellent method to starve pathogens in the body while strengthening our immune health. The imbalance of pathogens are often the root cause of many inflammatory flare-ups in the body. The pathogens love to feed off of inflammatory foods, then not only will they proliferate and flourish, they will basically poop. This toxic waste, along with many other toxins such as pesticides, chemicals, etc, causes our lymphatic system to become overwhelmed. So, this protocol gives our body and immune system a fighting chance to catch up and be in charge again, while calming and soothing at the same time.

Although this diet is very straight-forward and simple, it can be a challenge to shift old, negative patterns in our eating habits. We can frame this reset as granting a gift to ourselves for better health and the potential to bring profound awareness to the fact that we may have been living in a low quality of life that could be easily improved with some small choices.

There are no shortcuts or blood tests that are more accurate than a proper elimination & reintroduction protocol. And in prospective, out of the big picture of our entire life, it's only a blink in time that we need to set aside. The rewards of improved energy & well-being will undoubtedly outweigh
the effort.

My personal experience

In my personal past experience with fighting chronic health issues, I was also stubborn and didn't want to change my diet. I'm a foodie with a culinary degree! But, I also couldn't ignore how badly I would feel after eating certain foods. Without being aware of a diet like this one, I took years and years, slowly eliminating foods one by one with no significant change to my health. Once I was finally desperate enough and I was sick & tired of being sick & tired, I found this diet. I maintained the promise to myself to stick to it for 30 days and to correctly & patiently re-enter the foods back in. There were foods that I already knew didn't love me back the way I loved them (like gluten & dairy), so I didn't bother inviting them back.

Two weeks into the first 30 days of the elimination diet, my pain and inflammation faded away, my energy levels dramatically increased, my digestion improved and my fear of eating due to the rashes & hives it sometimes caused, began to dissipate. That of course gave me the motivation to complete the diet but it continues still today on the food choices I make. I now know exactly what foods work for my body and what works against me.

There were definitely foods that I was surprised to react to - ones that I ate almost everyday. While I was sad about needing to exclude those from my daily diet, I felt a sense of great empowerment that I was now in control of how my body felt.

I went two years straight strictly avoiding the foods that triggered me and for my personal case, that was what was needed to push me across the line from sick and maintaining to well & thriving. My lifestyle requires me to have a high amount of energy and I understand what it takes to maintain & create that energy in my body. Now, I stick to a very clean, low inflammatory type of diet for breakfast, lunch & dinner for 5-6 days per week and if I want to go out to a fabulous restaurant and indulge once per week - I do! If I ordered a great meal that IS inflammatory, I do my best to enjoy that meal in the moment because taking the leftovers home to expose my body to it a second time is not a wise choice.

When the people around you give you a hard time for making loving choices for your body & health, take it as a compliment. They might not be used to this strong new version of you. The common challenge would be my loved ones saying that I was being picky & ridiculous and that I don't like a food anymore and that certainly was NOT the case. I LOVE food and beverages but not all food & beverage loves me back.
The choice to respect your body in this way, is one of the highest expressions of self-love.

How to get started:

- Check out the "Foods to Avoid" list & strictly remove ALL of these foods for the first 30 days. Once you get to 30 days, you can decide if you need to extend to 60 or even 90 days of complete elimination.

- Check out the "Foods to Include" list and start making your grocery list and meal plans. Keep it simple.

- During the first 30 days, take note of how you feel.
    - increased energy?
    - less brain fog?
    - less pain & inflammation?
    - more endurance?
    - better digestion?
    - improved mood?

- Once you get to the 30 day mark and you have noted that all inflammatory related issues have subsided, you can move to the next phase. If issues are still present, stick to the full elimination for up to 90 days. Be patient with your body's healing process.

- Next phase is the re-introduction phase. Do not rush this phase. There are many resources on the different methods for reintroduction and for what to add back in first and for how long to wait in between introducing the next food.Decide what resonates with you.

- Final Phase is to incorporate your new personalized diet into your life. You will now know what foods trigger reactions and you can decide what is worth having on occasion and what is not.

Inflammatory Foods to Avoid:

All Additives
All Alcohol
All Eggs

Dairy
Butter
Cream
Cheese
Ghee
Milk
Yogurt

Gluten & Grains
Amaranth
Barley
Buckwheat
Bulger
Corn
Millet
Oats
Quinoa
Rice (all)
Sorghum
Spelt
Wheat

Legumes
Black Beans
Chickpeas
Cocoa (chocolate)
Fava Beans
Kidney Beans
Lentils
Lima Beans
Peanut
Soy Beans

Nightshades
Eggplant
Goji Berries
Ground Cherry
Peppers
 (Bell, Chili, Paprika,
Cayenne)
Red Spices (all)
Potato
Tobacco
Tomato

ALL SUGAR
(Natural sugars like
honey, maple syrup &
coconut sugar are ok
on occasion in
moderation)

Nuts/Seeds/
Spices
& some Oils
Almond
Brazil Nut
Canola
Cashew
Chia
Coffee
Cocoa
Flax
Hazelnut
Hemp
Pecan
Pine Nuts
Pistachio
Pumpkin
Safflower
Sesame
Sunflower
Walnut

Nourishing Foods to Include:

Vegetables
Artichoke
Arugula
Asparagus
Beets
Broccoli
Brussel Sprouts
Bok Choy
Cabbage
Carrots
Cauliflower
Chard
Cucumber
Fennel
Jicama
Kale
Leek
Lettuce
Mushroom
Onion
Parsnip
Rutabaga
Spinach
Squash
Sweet Potato

Fruits
Apple
Apricot
Avocado
Banana
Berries
Cherries
Citrus
Coconut
Date
Fig
Grapes
Kiwi
Mango
Melons
Peach
Pear
Persimmon
Plum
Pineapple
Pomegranate
Watermelon

Fats
Avocado Oil
Beef Tallow
Chicken Fat
Coconut Oil
Olive Oil
Palm Oil

Herbs & Spices
Basil
Bay Leaf
Chives
Cilantro
Cinnamon
Dill
Ginger
Garlic
Mint
Parsley
Peppermint
Rosemary
Saffron
Sage
Thyme
Tumeric

Proteins
Beef
Bison
Chicken
Duck
Fish
Lamb
Shellfish
Turkey
Venison

Pantry
Apple Cider
 Vinegar
Arrowroot
 Starch
Carob
 Powder
Cassava
 Flour
Coconut
 Flour
Coconut
 Sugar
Dried Fruit
Honey
Tapioca
 Starch
Tigernut
 Flour

Green Tea
Matcha
Black Tea
(Caffeine in
moderation)
Herbal Teas

Creating a daily ritual

When we include something new into our routine and pair it with powerful intention, we create a ritual for ourselves. Intentions can turn a boring daily checklist into small, individual, sacred rituals that can elevate our life experience.

A few intentions I visualize:

- Imagine the body as a beautiful, sacred temple
- Bring awareness to the vital life forces flowing through our bodies.
- Bring our attention to the present moment.

Powerful intention setting includes writing our intentions down. Doing this brings more importance to self care. Mapping out our new rituals in a daily, weekly or monthly calendar creates a promise to ourselves.

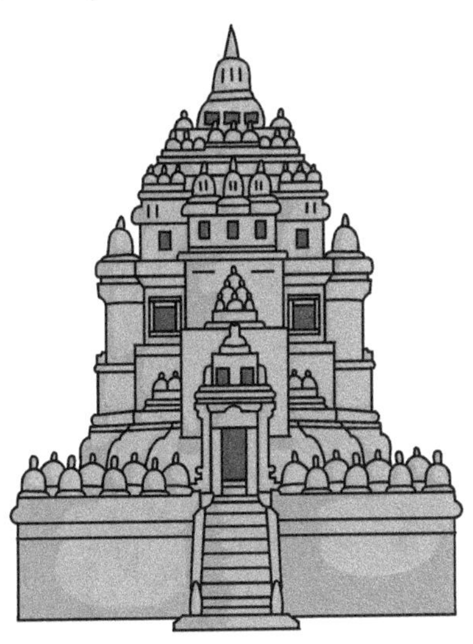

DO SOMETHING TODAY THAT YOUR FUTURE SELF WILL THANK YOU FOR.

Our actions and decisions today will shape the way we will be living in the future.

Conclusion

Beginning a healthy lymphatic lifestyle can be as simple as breathing & hydrating and as enjoyable to maintain as a cup of hot matcha and a sacred bath. The more challenging tips will be the most rewarding and the result is a journey to optimal health that can be felt within the first 30 days.

I'm so excited to invite you to join in on living a lymphatic lifestyle of your own. Map out one week at a time of what tips you'd like to start including and when & how you will make the time & space each day. Journaling this in a daily, weekly & monthly planner will help keep us accountable and give us a clear vision of the goals we want to accomplish. At the end of each day or week, acknowledge your wins, as well as, what you'd like to improve upon.

Please visit the website and take advantage of the FREE printable food lists & planning sheets at:

www.LaurelWestLMT.com

DAILY RITUALS

WEEK OF _______________

MORNING RITUALS	M	T	W	T	F	S	S

AFTERNOON RITUALS	M	T	W	T	F	S	S

EVENING RITUALS	M	T	W	T	F	S	S

www.LaurelWestLMT.com

DAILY PLANNER

DATE: /   /

07:00

08:00

09:00

10:00

11:00

12:00

13:00

14:00

15:00

16:00

17:00

18:00

19:00

20:00

21:00

REMINDERS

SHOPPING LIST

MEALS

WATER INTAKE

MOOD TRACKER

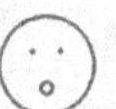

www.LaurelWestLMT.com

WEEKLY HABIT TRACKER

DATE: / /

MORNING ROUTINE

	M	T	W	T	F	S	S

HEALTH + WELLNESS

	M	T	W	T	F	S	S

SELF-CARE + WELLBEING

	M	T	W	T	F	S	S

EVENING ROUTINE

	M	T	W	T	F	S	S

RITUAL CHECKLIST

SAMPLE

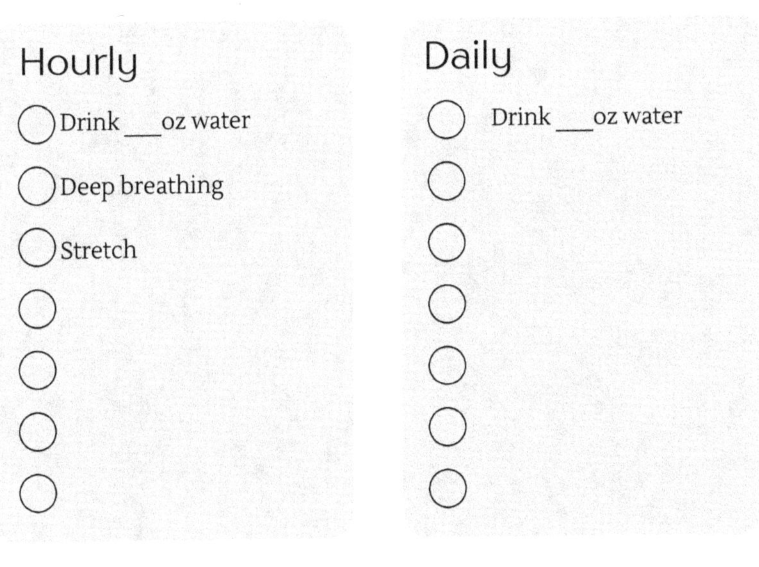

www.LaurelWestLMT.com

About the Author

Laurel is a licensed manual therapist, specializing in Holistic Wellness, Advanced Lymph Drainage Therapy & Cranio-Sacral Therapy and is a Master Energy Healing Practitioner. She has been practicing Lymphatic Massage since 2012. Her experience includes thousands of hands-on sessions with a wide array of clients with therapeutic needs ranging from: post-surgery, oncology, "auto-immune" symptoms, digestive distress, sinus congestion, allergies, toxin exposure, chronic headaches, PTSD, neuro-inflammations, chronic fatigue and much more.

Laurel's Advanced Lymph Drainage training is from Dr. Bruno Chikly of The Chikly Institute. Advanced Lymphatic addresses not only the superficial lymph system that is skin deep, but also the deep pathways, lymphatic of the muscles, fascia, viscera (organs), brain (glymphatic) and more.

Being a Master Energy Healing Practitioner, allows her to be highly attuned to all energy flow, rhythms & balance or the lack thereof. This natural ability to feel energy movement in and around a client's body combined with extensive training from brilliant teachers, mentors, peers and clients has molded her into the therapist she is today.

Laurel currently resides in Georgetown, TX and has lived in the Austin, TX area since early childhood.

She enjoys spending time with her family, friends and her beloved dog, Luke, as well as, spending time outdoors in nature, cooking and exploring new restaurants, listening to music. She is constantly expanding & learning more about alternative health, holistic wellness, culinary medicine, herbal medicine, energy medicine & cosmic energy.

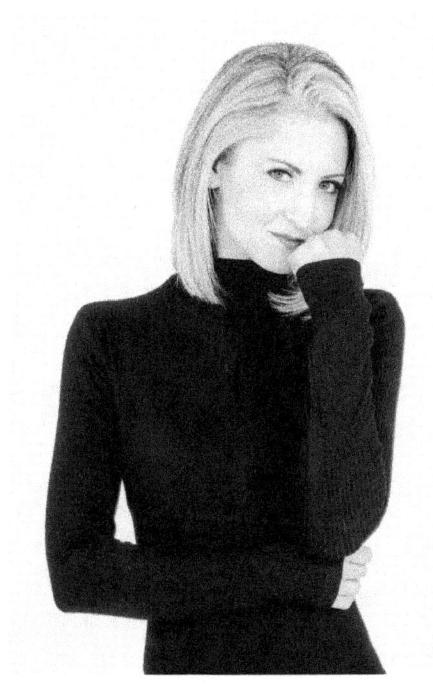

Wishing you optimal health,
happiness & longevity.

Laurel West, LMT

Thank you for reading!

Thank you so much for purchasing this book. If you found any of these tips helpful, please consider recommending this book to a friend or loved one and leaving an excellent review on Amazon.

Connect with Laurel:

Instagram: @LaurelWestLMT

www.Laurelwestlmt.com